797,885 Books
are available to read at

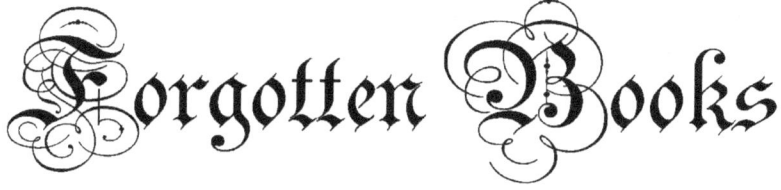

www.ForgottenBooks.com

Forgotten Books' App
Available for mobile, tablet & eReader

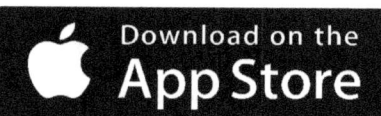

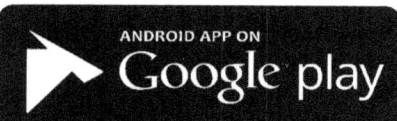

ISBN 978-1-334-52448-6
PIBN 10704604

This book is a reproduction of an important historical work. Forgotten Books uses
state-of-the-art technology to digitally reconstruct the work, preserving the original format
whilst repairing imperfections present in the aged copy. In rare cases, an imperfection in
the original, such as a blemish or missing page, may be replicated in our edition. We do,
however, repair the vast majority of imperfections successfully; any imperfections that
remain are intentionally left to preserve the state of such historical works.

Forgotten Books is a registered trademark of FB &c Ltd.
Copyright © 2017 FB &c Ltd.
FB &c Ltd, Dalton House, 60 Windsor Avenue, London, SW19 2RR.
Company number 08720141. Registered in England and Wales.

For support please visit www.forgottenbooks.com

1 MONTH OF FREE READING

at

www.ForgottenBooks.com

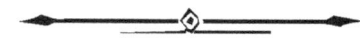

By purchasing this book you are eligible for one month membership to ForgottenBooks.com, giving you unlimited access to our entire collection of over 700,000 titles via our web site and mobile apps.

To claim your free month visit:

www.forgottenbooks.com/free704604

* Offer is valid for 45 days from date of purchase. Terms and conditions apply.

English
Français
Deutsche
Italiano
Español
Português

www.forgottenbooks.com

Mythology Photography **Fiction**
Fishing Christianity **Art** Cooking
Essays Buddhism Freemasonry
Medicine **Biology** Music **Ancient Egypt** Evolution Carpentry Physics
Dance Geology **Mathematics** Fitness
Shakespeare **Folklore** Yoga Marketing
Confidence Immortality Biographies
Poetry **Psychology** Witchcraft
Electronics Chemistry History **Law**
Accounting **Philosophy** Anthropology
Alchemy Drama Quantum Mechanics
Atheism Sexual Health **Ancient History**
Entrepreneurship Languages Sport
Paleontology Needlework Islam
Metaphysics Investment Archaeology
Parenting Statistics Criminology
Motivational

BORCK, E.

DIAGNOSIS OF
OVARIAN TUMORS.

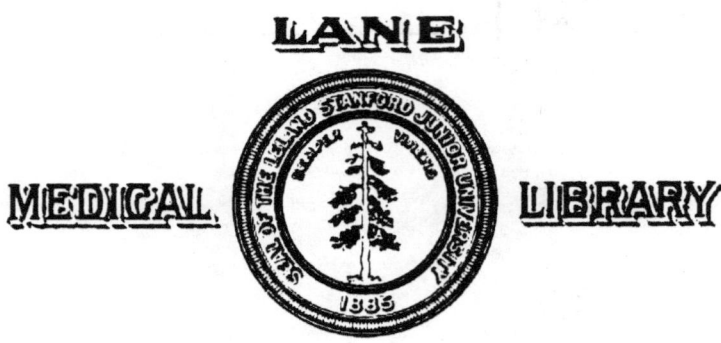

DIAGNOSIS

OV R   MORS.

LECTURES DELIVERED BY

EDW. BORCK, A. M., M. D.

PROFESSOR OF SURGERY, ETC., ETC.

ST. LOUIS, MO.
C. M. Curtman, Print, 710 N. Third Street

PREFACE.

These lectures were delivered during the first three sessions of 1882-83, at the College for Medical Practitioners, St. Louis, Mo. Published at the request of many professional friends near and distant, who were not able to listen to me in person. I prepared the first part for the Cincinnati Obstetrical Gazette, wherein it appeared in September, 1883.

This reprint, with additional tables, and my method of operating, is dedicated to the class of Medical Practitioners who attended my lectures during the above named sessions.

BY THE AUTHOR.

LECTURE XIV.
Diagnosis of Ovarian Tumors.

GENTLEMEN!

In our last lecture we considered abdominal tumors in general, and studied the various modes by which we are enabled to make a correct diagnosis, and under that head included also hernias. To-day we will take up a class of tumors to which that fair sex, whom we all adore and love so much, alone is heir to, Ovarian Tumors.

And as I speak to men that have had years of experience in their profession and love their study, I take it for granted that you are all acquainted with the pathology—I need not occupy your time with repeating what you can read. As usual, you find a roster upon the wall, which will inform you of the papers and articles lately written upon that subject. In addition I call your attention to this little work of Garrigue's, which I received a little while ago. Let us consider the diagnosis and take a simple case of ovarian tumor for our guide. It matters not what kind of an ovarian tumor we have, so we know it is ovarian and nothing else, and do not mistake it for other tumors or swellings or the reverse.

For convenience sake, the development of an ovarian tumor may be divided into four stages. Now let me make a diagram: on the left side the tumor begins to grow; as long as it is within the pelvis it is in the first stage; if it grows up to the umbilicus, it is in the second stage; from here to epigastrium, it is in the third stage; and up to its highest point. In the fourth stage its prominence and circumference is alone increased. Between those boundry lines you may make subdivisions again if you choose. The reason why these tumors occur more upon the left side, is owing to the fact that the left ovarian veins have no valves.

Now let us reflect for a moment and see what disturbance we may expect to be produced by such a growth.

In the first stage: If the uterus is in a normal position, the tumor is behind the uterus and in front of the bladder. There is irritation of the bladder, dysmenorrhœa, constipation, a feeling of a heaviness in the pelvis and hemorrhoids, the latter being frequent with polycysts.

In the second stage: What must it do? It must displace the small intestines to the opposite side, and as it has arisen out of the pelvis the uterus is therefore placed behind the cyst, and the bladder goes with the uterus. The tumor by this time has acquired a pedicle and is movable, the patient discovers it rolling about as a ball, if no adhesion has been formed. There is a desire to urinate, but diminished action of the kidneys.

In the third stage: The small intestines are pushed up, the large omentum is only between the tumor and the abdominal walls, it is up to the epigastrum, presses upon the stomach and diaphragm, elevates the ribs, interferes with respiration and digestion, produces palpitation of the heart, and the general health fails. We have derangements of menstruation, emaciation of face and neck and upper extremities. There is a peculiar expression of the countenance, enlargement of the abdominal veins and œdema of the lower extremeties.

In the fourth stage: The tumor extends in all directions where there is no resistance, all the symptoms are aggravated, the pulse runs up to 120-130.

I make these preliminary remarks to refresh your memory. Now suppose a patient comes to us with symptoms like these:—her abdomen has increased gradually in volume, without any sickness; she tells us the swelling first appeared in the iliac region and extended upwards; she has also observed in the beginning of the growth, by turning quickly in bed, a feeling like a ball rolling about her abdomen. If the swollen abdomen appears like an advanced pregnancy, with well and equal fluctuation. if there is a dull sound in the anterior abdominal region in every position, but on the side a tympanitic sound upon percussion, if by the motions we impart to the swelling the uterus moves along but is of normal depth, then we can suspect an ovarian cyst. The whole character of the swelling speaks in favor of a cyst, the passive movements of the uterus along with the tumor indicates that the tumor belongs to the internal generative organs. The passive movements produced with the uterus and the normal size of the same, indicates to us that the swelling does not belong to the uterus; it must be an ovarian cyst. And we can prove this positively by making examination per rectum—and here I will say to you, make your examinations always for healthy organs, do not hunt for an ovarian cyst, but for two normal ovaries—if you find both in their physiological condition, exclude disease of the ovary, the swelling must be something else. If you find but one ovary normal, and the other mentioned symptoms in addition, you will not go amiss to say ovarian tumor.

Aspiration of the fluid and the chemical and microscopical examination will clear up any doubt. The chemical character is principally albumen, extractive matters, fat and salt united with water, but it contains no fibrin, and the fluid is not spontaneously coaguable. (Here the microscopical appearance of what the fluid reveals, was shown, after Drysdale.) Now after this you may think it easy to make a correct diagnosis, but be not deceived, it is sometimes very difficult. Let me relate to you, the history of a case. An American lady 25 years old, married, had two children, one living, 5 years old, she informed me when I first saw her in consultation with the physician then in attendance. that three years previously she noticed a swelling in her left iliac region, which gradually grew larger; she felt that something was rolling about in her abdomen. She kept it secret and at last she became so large, that her friends thought her pregnant with twins or triplets. She had suffered all this time with intermittent fever. Six months previous, she had gone north and came home improved in health. Physicians had recommended tapping, but it was not resorted to. She had passed a good deal of water at times, could not tell exactly, but believed it came from the bladder, then became more natural in size, still a large lump remained. The last three months she grew worse, the swelling became hard, every sixth day she would have anattack of fever and pain in abdomen. " Inflammatory attack, Peritonitis."

When I first saw this patient, and before knowing anything about her particulars of the history of the case, I ventured to say to the attending physician, that I expected to find an ovarian cyst, simply by the characteristic expression of the face. Upon an examination, I found a large tumor in the left side, extending up to the umbilicus. Near the umbilicus a distinct fluctuation, which I recognized as an abscess, or possibly nature's effort to open in that region; adhesion only on right side and in front of tumor, left lower side none, I could lift up the abdominal muscles there. Fluctuation otherwise not distinct, the whole tumor somewhat movable, uterus normal, and pushed to right side. Per vagina tumor could be felt; per rectum, right ovary plain, left not detectable, but tumor distinct. Great irritability of the stomach. She had been seen by a host of physicians, some eminent and well known, but no opinion was given; that is no one committed himself to a positive diagnosis. Poultices, liniment, etc., had been applied externally, also internal medication, all to no purpose. Only temporary relief was obtained; she was very weak, no cancerous cachexia, no family history of cancer. I diagnosed positive a ovarian tumor, but gave a guarded opinion in regard to complications, recommended a tonic regimen to build her up. She recruited nicely. When I saw her again ten days later I was informed that she had passed something like fluid and matter, amounting to a quart, from her bowels. She was anxious to have something done to relieve her suffering. I recommended an operation, and carefully stated to all concerned, that I would make an exploratory incision and then if advisable go on with the operation, otherwise abandon it. They all gladly consented in good hopes.—Now what do you expect? After opening the abdomen, I found a whole mass of adhesion, omentum, mesentery, intestines, all adherent together to the abdominal walls; the abdominal walls cancerous; the fluctuation we detected near the umbilicus turned out to be an encysted abscess; while cutting through the abdomen in the linia albae, a crackling sound could be heard; no where could an opening be found, all was one mass of adhesion. My assistants all looked at me, and I felt like I had made a mistake, or that I had been deceived in my diagnosis. I could not apprehend that I was mistaken finally I succeeded in getting my finger between the walls of the abdomen, and hunted for the left ovary. I assure you I felt relieved and confess, a little proud, when I exhibited a plain tumor, of that ovary about as large as a French turnip, a shriveled up sac without fluid. I could peel it out of the surrounding cancerous mass.

The patient's fate was sealed, but it was an instructive case—an ovarian cyst, which nature had tried to cure spontaneously, and a development of malignant growth not from the tumor, but from other parts and from other unknown causes, surrounding, or better, enveloping the tumor. They are perplexing cases! Not one symptom alone, but all combined should be taken into consideration and carefully studied and weighed.

It is said of Thomas Keith, that he did not make a single mistake in his diagnosis in 200 successive cases. I can not say this, because my cases have not yet run up to that number. But I can say, that in all my own cases, and in those which I have examined for others, up to this time, I have been fortunate enough. My diagnosis has always been verified. In regard to my success, I prefer others to inform you.

Pregnancy, encysted dropsy of the peritoneum, uterine fibroid tumors, distended bladder, renal tumors and cysts, cysts of the broad ligament, (these by the way are considered as the most difficult to diagnose,) ascites., etc., etc., have all been, and may again be mistaken for ovarian tumors. Again, ovarian cysts may be complicated with pregnancy, ascites, uterine fibroma and second cyst.

Ascites is mistaken the most frequently for ovarian dropsy, though that mistake ought not to be made by any practitioner.

In ascites the intestine floats upon the fluid, consequently in the recumbent position of the patient, the dull sound must be heard at the lowest point, the tympanitic sounds upon the highest point of the abdomen. In ovarian cyst the reverse. If the patient change her position in ascites, the fluid will always gravitate to the lowest point, the intestine floating upon it. In ovarian cyst it remains the same. It is also well to remember that œdema of the extremities appears after tumor is developed, but often precedes it in ascites. As I have said to you of other surgical affections, that it is not well nor prudent for the surgeon at once to go to work with his hands and feel and twist and pinch the parts injured, but should first of all inspect with his eyes; and educate them as perfectly as possible to observe the different outlines; always having in his brain the normal contours and position, and then mark the abnormal. Here we can learn a good deal to our advantage with the aid of our eyes, look at these drawings.

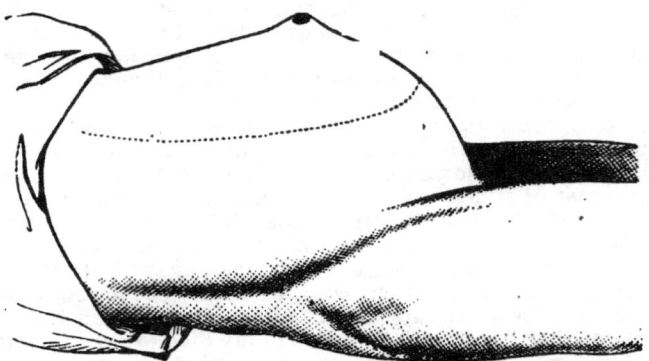

FIG. 1 is a lateral view of the abdomen affected with ascites.

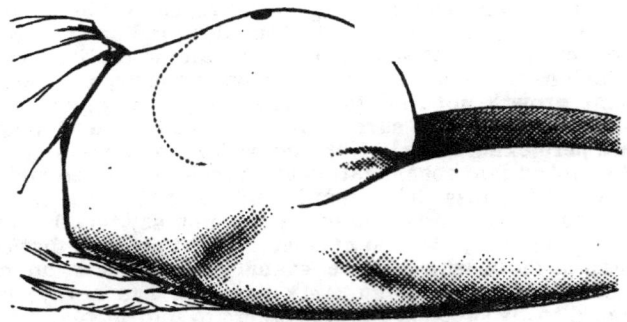

FIG. 2 is a lateral view of the abdomen affected with an ovarian cyst.
(*Albert.*)

We can see at once the difference in the shape and out-lines, it needs no explanation. Observe the difference between the sternum and the umbilicus, and pubis, and look at the umbilicus itself, it may be obliterated in ovarian dropsy, but never presents an arching like it does in ascites, etc. One point I wish to call your attention to in ovarian cyst, you can grasp the abdominal wall between your fingers and lift them up from the tumor, where ever there is no adhesion; in ascites you can not do it.

The symptoms and signs of pregnancy I need not explain to you, you understand them too well, but let us remember that in the patient affectted with an ovarian cyst the breast may become enlarged, and an areola around the nipples may be present, also morning sickness.

Of the diagnosis of uterine fibroid tumors, you will hear all about that from the Professor of gynæcology, in the course of his lectures.

In regard to a distended bladder, all I wish to say is this: never under any circumstances depend upon the nurse or even the patient herself; they may be honest in telling you that she had just passed water, and a good deal of it. I lately met with a case and received such information, yet I introduced the catheter and draw off a large amount of urine, I do this every time before examining. Recollect the case on record related to you of a child where the urethra was closed and the bladder adhered to the umbilicus and at or near that place, was a fistulous opening, where from the urine dribbled; She was operated upon at the age of 18 years, and a passage made at the natural situation; the fistulous opening closed spontaneously. We meet sometimes with adhesion of the bladder at that point, as a complication with ovarian cyst. Again, there are cases on record where an ovarian cyst became adherent to the umbilicus, and formed a fistulous opening and a spontaneous cure took place.

How to diagnose tumors and cysts of the kidney. I have already spoken to you in a previous lecture; do not forget that tumors of the kidneys will enlarge from the posterior to the anterior part above; and they push the intestine in front. The colon here is always in front and can be filled with air and be distended thereby and recognized.

In the cyst of the broad ligament, the fluid is always as clear as spring water, contains no albumen; and a manual examination per rectum under chloroform, will detect two ovaries. These are the cytss that are cured by tapping.

Now this drawing represents a side view of an abdomen affected with a multilocular cyst, and this is a portrait of the characteristic feature (facies ovariana, after Wells) The time of one hour is too short to go into details about everything, but to do you and the subject justice, I have prepared these tables, you see hanging upon the walls, which you may study for yourselves. See tables, pages 9 and 10.

Here you have the differential diagnosis of a mono cyst, a poly cyst and a dermoid cyst.

Then here the chemical consistence of the fluids of an ovarian cyst, cyst of the broad ligament, amniotic fluid, and ascitic fluid. And here what the microscope reveals.

All this will give you a pretty good idea of the difficulties we may encounter, and what is necessary to make a correct diagnosis; and inconclusion I will say to you again: Be systematic in all your doings; only by following and carrying out a certain system, can we expect to come any ways near to perfection. Let me repeat then:

Take first the symptoms into consideration, the history of the case, the expression of the face and neck, the activity of the kidneys, the sympathetic affections of the mammæ; then the local signs; the rationae as detected by the patient; then the physical local signs; exploration, such as, inspection, menstruation, palpitation, percussion, auscultation, change of position, vaginal touch, trocar, microscope; and last of all exploratory incision.

Second: Ask yourselves the following questions, so beautifully illustrated by the late Dr. Peasle, and answer each and every one of them positively, viz.:

Is there actually an enlargement within the cavity?

Is there fluctuation, indicating an accumulation of fluid within the abdomen, or a solid tumor? "Mesenteric fibroma or fibro-plastic."

Is the fluctuation due to ascites?

Does the cause of the enlargement arise in the pelvis?

Is not the tumor a pregnant tumor?

Is there not still an enlargement of the uterus though it be not gravid? "Hæmatometra, hydrometra, uterine hypertrophy, fibroma, carcinoma of fundus, uterine fibro cysts."

And to what is the fluctuation due? Serous cyst of the broad ligament, encysted dropsy of periotoneum, dropsy of fallopian tubes, renal cyst hepatic cyst, pelvic abscess, splinic abscess, etc."

In our next lecture we will take up the treatment, or rather when and how to operate, and I will demonstrate to you my method of operating.

OVARIAN DROPSY.	ASCITES.
The tumor is most prominent upon one side, save in advanced stages.	The tumor is uniform and symmetrical.
The tumor remains prominent and globular in all positions of the body.	The tumor *flattens* and *increases in its breadth* on lying down.
The tumor is locally fluctuant.	The tumor fluctuates through the *entire abdomen*.
The tumor begins in one iliac fossa.	The tumor begins symmetrically from below.
The percussion is dull in front when the patient lies upon her back, but is tympanitic, from displaced intestine, at the sides.	The percussion is resonant in front of abdomen, when patient lies on the back, as the bowel floats; but is *flat* at the sides of the abdomen.
Is constant and not affected by attitude.	Is vairable, and is affected by attitudes of patient and by amount of fluid present.
Palpation detects an oval outline and an irregular surface to the tumor.	No circumscribed outline to tumor or irregularity of surface is discovered.
The cervix of uterus is normal in position.	The cervix is frequently displaced.
The health is generally good until the tumor becomes large.	The health is usually impaired from the commencement.
If present, œdema of the limbs *follows* the advent of tumor.	It often *precedes* the ascites.
Aortic pulsation *may* be transmitted.	Aortic pulsation is never present.
No apparent cause exists.	*Hepatic*, *cadiac*, or *renal* disease often co-exists.
Normal color and moisture of the skin exist.	The skin is often jaundiced, and is frequently dry like parchment.
Fluid drawn by aspirator reveals	*Ranney*.

OVARIAN FLUID.
(*Drysdale.*)

Microscope may reveals:
Epithelial cells; oil globules; granular matter; cholestrine; ovarian granular cells; blood cells; Pus cells; Gluge's inflammatory corpuscles.

ASCITES.

Microscope reveals:
Pus cells; oil globules; amoeboid bodies; squamous epithelium.

HEALTHY AMNITOIC

Is a thin, pale, straw-colored fluid, turbid and flocculi, has a peculiar odor—deposit occurs—on standing, its chemical character is alkaline, specific gravity: 1005-1010—contains no fibrin; but albumen, acid acet, clouds it, becomes opaque on boiling. Microscope reveals: Epithelial cells; small tesellated cells, with oil globules and flocculi. Aether dissolves the last.

FLUID DRAWN BY ASPIRATOR REVALS.

OVARIAN.	ASCITES.
Amber or brown color.	Light straw-colored.
Not spontaneously congulable.	Spontaneously congulable if fibrinous.
Specific gravity 1018 to 1024.	Specific gravity, 1010 to 1015.
Albumen and metalbumen.	

CYST OF BROAD LIGAMENT.	OVARIAN CYST — THIRD STAGE.
Very slow growth; rare; always monocystic.	Common; growth more rapid; two forms of cystoma.
Mostly in young persons.	Occurs at all ages.
Expression natural; not much emaciation.	Expression changed; emaciation.
General health slightly impaired — though in third stage.	Decidedly impaired.
Abdominal veins less prominent.	Veins more developed.
Fluctuation remarkably distinct.	Less distinct.
Uterus lies low, generally.	Not depressed, but behind tumor generally.
Per vaginam, fluctuation very clear.	Less clear.
Fluid contains no albumen, and is as clear as spring-water. (Specific gravity 1005.)	Contains much albumen, and is not perfectly transparent. (Specific gravity 1015 or more.)
Scarcely ever fills after tapping.	Fills again after tapping.
Very seldom fatal.	Almost always fatal at last.
	(*Peaslee.*)

MONOCYST.	POLYCYST.	DERMOID CYST.
Slower growth. Not common.	Rapid growth. More common.	Congenital. Very slow. Very rare.
Peculiar expression comes later.	Comes much earlier.	Latest of all.
General health fails much later.	Fails early; by end of second stage.	Very late.
Abdomen symmetrical; if monocyst salient, pointed.	Not symmetrical; not pointed.	Not symmetrical.
Enlargement from 35 to 45 inches.	Sometimes to 55 or even 78 inches.	Smallest; generally 30 to 40 inches.
Surface smooth if monocyst.	Lobulated; irregular.	A monocyst, as a rule.
Tumor disappears after tapping.	Does not disappear.	Does not completely collapse.
Œdema of lower extremities very rare; abdominal veins less enlarged and later.	Very common. Veins enlarged early.	Very uncommon.
Adhesions less common and less firm.	Adhesions the rule, and vascular.	Adhesions not very rare.
Inflammation of cyst-wall not common.	Not so common.	Most common, proportionally.
Ulceration of cyst-wall not common.	More common.	Most common of all.
Spontaneous rupture not common.	Far more common.	Very uncommon.
Amenorrhœa comes later.	Comes much earlier.	Very late.
Fluctuation distinct, and throughout if a monocyst; and from any point to all others.	Less distinct, and circumscribed.	Fluctuation more obscure.
Per vaginam, uterus is higher, and the fluctuation also.	Uterus lower, and the fluctuation also, or none at all.	Uterus lower; fluctuation dull.

Pedicle longer, as a rule. Fluid limpid, amber, bluish, or greenish, viscid, with much albumen. Contains epithelial scales, cholesterine, and fatty granules, and the ovarian glomeruli.	Shorter as a rule. Not clear, brownish, dense, gelatinous, or albuminous. Contains also blood-pigment and blood-corpuscles.	No rule. Light color, curdy, no albumen, partly soluble in either. Contains epithelial scales, sebaceous matter, crystals of cholesterine, hairs, etc., etc.; a single hair is pathognomonic.
Exception. — An oligocyst of but two or three constituent cysts, with thin partitions, may give all the signs of a monocyst.		

(*Peasle.*)

LECTURE XV.
Method of Operating.

GENTLEMEN!

We will now take up the operation and I will explain to you my method. We will take it for granted, that before proceeding with the operation, that you made a correct diagnosis and have prepared the patient in the very best condition, have given the evening before an enema to clear out the bowels, and allowed a cup of milk and bread. On the morning of the operation, have the patient bathed, dressed with a short gown, flannel drawers and stockings. Let her rest in an easy-chair, covered with a blanket, and if her skin is not moist, steam her with some hot water, or apply hot water bottles to her feet. This is essential; dry cold skin would be a disadvantage. Give her 10 gr. of quinine and $\frac{1}{4}$ gr. of morphine an hour before the operation. And by all means have her confidence fully, never persuade one to be operated on, but let the patient implore you to do so. At the same time your operating room, which should be the best room in the house, must have been prepared according to your own directions, and it is best to give them in writing or print as follows:

The room should be about 80^0 F. during the operation and kept at about at 70^0 F. afterwards. Free circulation of air should be secured.

All furniture, carpets, curtains, etc., are to be removed; the room is to be freshly whitewashed, floor and woodwork all scrubbed with soap and water, and rinsed with water and chlorinated soda, one to two tumblerfuls to a bucketful of soft water. Procure a small, new bed-lounge six feet long and twenty-eight inches broad, with two square blocks of wood six inches high, or more, with holes drilled into them to receive the rollers of the feet of the bed, to make it stand solid and firm, and to elevate the bed to a proper height to suit the operator. Have a good firm mattress to fit the bed it must be nine or ten inches high; two small tables; one chair; two yards of Indian rubber or oil cloth to spread over the bed; one-half dozen soft towels, three or four stone wash-bowls, and one pitcher; one thermometer; one clean bucket for water, and one cup; one old bucket or tub; tumblers, drinking water, tea spoon; three or four clean wooden hoops, and a bed-pan. The towels, as well as the bed clothes and dresses, must be well washed and rinsed in the solution of chlorinated soda; but not be starched. During the operation no one is allowed to leave or enter the room. Under no circumstances is any person permitted to visit the patient or remain in the room, except the nurse or the attending physician.

You should also see that the following is on hand, and give (in writing,) directions to the family **druggist.**

  ℞ Distilled Water......................5 gallons.
    Oil Silk..................................1 yard.
    Lister's Carbolized Gauze.......1 piece 5 yards.
    Alcohol................................ $\frac{1}{2}$ pint.
    Mitchell's Mole Skin Plaster............1 yard.
    Liq. Ferri. Persulphatis............... $\frac{1}{2}$ ounce.
    Brandy (French).......................1 pint.
    Pure Carbolic Acid....................1 ounce.
    Chloroform and Sulph. Ether each 1 pound.
    (Squibb's or Mallinckrodt's is best.)

Or Bichloride of Methyline, if the latter is used. I prefer Mallinckrodt's. I used it in several cases given through Jounker's apparatus, and it acts very nicely. Nevertheless I like the chloroform the best.

Nitrate of Methyl one drachm, is well to have on hand, and a Battery.

   R Iodine............................gr. ii.
     Pot. Jod..........................ʒ ss.
     Aquae Dest......................ʒ viii. M.

Sig. Use to fumigate the room before operation.

Here is the atomizer (Liston's spray). I will light it for you and you can observe how it works.

In my earlier operations, I used the carbolized spray during the operation. I now discard that plan as not necessary.

   R Acid Carbolic....................ʒ ss.
     Glycerinae......................ʒ vii. ss. M.

Sig. Ready to be mixed with water to wash the hands, instruments and sponges. The sponges should be new, and of the finest quality; previously well washed in a weak solution of Nitric Acid, then kept in carbolized water.

   R Acid Carbolic....................ʒ i.
     Oli Olive........................ʒvi. M.

Sig. Used to pour upon a saucer or plate; the ligatures and threaded needles are laid and kept in this until needed.

   R Chloride of Sodium..............ʒiv.
     Albumen..........................ʒvi.
     Distilled Water..................oi. M.

Sig.: Used for dipping in the hands, instruments and sponges, after disinfection, and before using them (this is the artificial serum) and has to be diluted with three parts of warm water, the temperature of blood heat. It is also used to syringe out the abdominal cavity, to clean it of any blood or fluid it may contain.

   R Pulv. Opii.........................
     Sacc. Albae.....................aa gr. xii.
     Misce et div. in Chart..........No. xii.

Sig.: Used as directed or needed.

   R Morph. Sulph...................gr. i.
     Aquae Dest.....................gtt C. M.

Sig.: For hypodermic injections.

"Listerine" may be well substituted for Carbolic Acid.

(All prescriptions should be marked in full on every bottle and package.)

So far your drugs and dressings. Now the **Instruments** I brought down my case, and will explain to you as I go along. Here is a plain trocar, ½-inch calibre, about 12 inches long, which I employ for tapping a cyst without further operation. It seems to be very large, but it is not; I first cut through the skin and cellular tissue with a scalpel, then introduce the trocar and draw off the fluid. The opening will contract almost completely. Here is another trocar like the Dome trocar, used for tapping a cyst after opening the abdominal cavity; you see it can be withdrawn and has a safety tube, and you can do no injury in searching for a partition within a cyst. This is a Dawson's Modified Clamp. Two wire retractors, three Peasle's needles, one tooth-edged scissors, one pair curved small scissors, one pair straight small scissors, one steel sound No. 10, for locating adhesions, one artery forceps slide catch, one female catheter, one pair wire cutting forceps, one steel grooved director, one arge tenaculum, one scalpel—fixed handle, one straight bistoury—fixed handle, one probe pointed bistoury — fixed handle, one artery needle — fixed handle, one dozen steel ovariotomy pins, one catgut ligature jar, one granite enameled iron tray, for carbolized silk or linen ligature, oil paper, oil pasteboard strips, etc; with room for needles, beads, iron and silver wire, etc. Here are two of my dressing and needle forceps, with slide catch six inches long, extra deep serrated.

These are my cyst elevators, made of strong steel wire, shaped like a tuning-fork, or lady's hair-pin, slightly curved, a double needle; and here is a cautery iron, and two pieces of rubber tubing about four feet long, one of them is fastened to the trocar. Also twenty-five or thirty fine needles ready threaded with fine linen ligatures, in case you should need them to stitch up any openings in the intestines or bladder that may happen to give away.

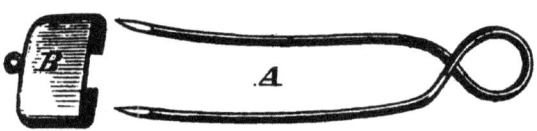

FIG. 1.— Half the smallest size.
A — The Elevator.   B — A cap to protect the points.

These are the instruments necessary for the operation. Have them all arranged conveniently upon a small table; see yourself that everything is in perfect order, and nothing missing, keep everything out of sight of the patient. Before your patient is brought in, arrange and designate the duties of each of your assistants, tell each of them what you expect him to do, and to do that and nothing else; place your main assistant on the left of the patient; one for the chloroform, who must be aware of his responsible duty. Intrust your sponges but to one person only, count them out to him, and before closing the abdomen, demand them all; see also that none of the instruments are missing, and allow no one to do anything, especially not, to put his hand into the abdomen, except you ask him to do so. One, ready for any emergency that may happen.

Do not talk, keep quiet and tranquil; have no lookers-on. And let me tell you, see that you have the very best of assistants, one superior to yourself is preferable, at least, equal; your main assistant should *never* be inferior to yourself, if possible. For one who knows and is acquainted with the operation will render you better service; be not afraid of him who has had the experience, for he was once there where you now begin, and he will act forbearingly with you. But avoid the one who is selfish, one who thinks he knows it all. An operator who for his own vanity's sake never employs any but ignorant nurses or young students, and others whom he can blindfold, and who will not be aware of and are not able to observe his mistakes, so that he may shine and appear to be a great light, will never gain a great success.

Everything being ready, the patient is brought in, laid upon the bed, covered, and chloroformed. The assistant will gently support the abdomen with his expanded hands. You begin your incision through the skin, a little below the umbilicus in the Linea Albae and carry it down to the pubis, then divide the cellular and adipose tissue, using your groove director, layer after layer, until you come to the peritoneal covering; if you miss the median line, move your director from side to side, and you will find it again. However, I think there is no harm, perhaps an advantage in cutting through the rectus muscle. Having reached the peritoneum, stop and wait until all hæmorrahge has ceased, Then pick up the peritoneal layer with a forceps, nick with the knife, and divide it the whole length. The cyst will now be exposed. You can recognize it by its bluish appearance; if you are not sure, examine it closely, you will see whether there are any adhesions, and may use the sound for that purpose. If you have not room enough, lengthen your incision. Having satisfied yourself about that, the next step will be to empty the cyst.

Let us suppose this bladder which lies before us, and which is filled with water, to be a cyst. You take the elevator and introduce it thus: See Fig. 2. Now take the trocar, thrust it into the cyst, between the prongs and fingers. See Fig. 3. The advantage of this method is: no fluid can escape from the cyst, and the sack empties itself; it is gently and very slowly drawn out, the trocar is pushed gently deeper at the same time; the abdominal walls collapsing around the cyst, which are supported by the hands of an assistant, thus preventing any of the viscera from protruding, and by the time the cyst is nearly empty, it is also almost drawn out from its bed; the hold is firm and unnecessary traction and manipulation is avoided and no air can enter. If needed a ligature can be applied around the cyst and trocar below the prongs of the elevator. With a little care all soiling of clothes and bedding can be prevented. This elevator may also be conveniently employed to transfix the pedicle, used with the ligature; with the cap in its place, the pedicle can be fixed in lower part of wound, the elevator resting transversely upon the outside of the abdomen, and no clamp at all is needed.

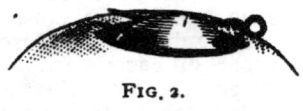

FIG. 2.

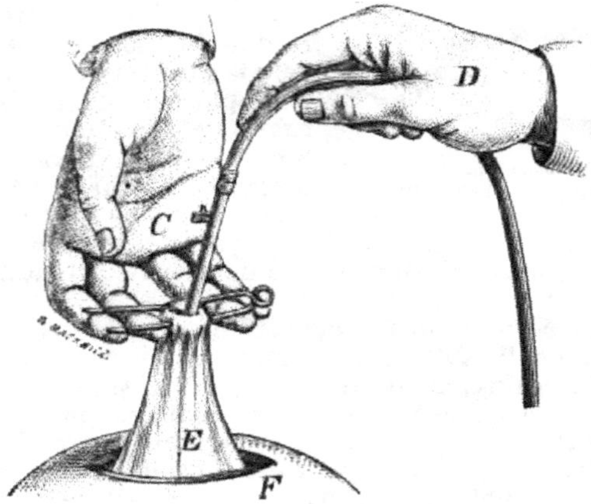

FIG. 3.
C—Right Hand of Assistant. D—Right Hand of Operator. E—The Cyst. F—Abdomen.

You see how nicely it works, it acts like a siphon, the thinnest cyst can be held in this way without tearing; the patient may be turned over on her side to facilitate matters. I have employed this method in all my operations except the first, this idea struck me then, and this little instrument has given me a great deal of pleasure, for a description of the same has appeared in many medical journals here and abroad, and has been been translated in almost all of the modern language. I may say it travelled around the globe.

The cyst now being emptied, adhesion if there are any, separated and bloodvessels tied, the whole mass lifted out of the abdomen, you take this clamp and secure the pedicle, and cut it off above the clamp with the serrated scissors. Now you must tie and secure the pedicle, always do this by transfixion, thus: Take one of these Peasle needles armed with a strong ligature, secured into handle, pushed through the middle of the pedicle, then slip in not less than 4 single strong silk threads, never roll them up rope-like, you can not secure a safe knot in that way. Now withdraw the needle with the silk, you have 4 ends on each side. Tie each half with two of the ligatures and the whole again with the other two, cut the ends short, now remove your clamps slowly, be sure that all bleeding has stopped.

By this time your cautery iron is ready heated to a black heat, clean it, and scorch the end of the pedicle, carefully, that is to say amalgamate it. Done! drop it into the pelvic cavety. The pedicle may also be treated without the cantery. It seems to me that instead of dividing the pedicle, it would be just as well to cut through the cyst close to the pedicle, leaving a part of the cyst upon the stump for protection, of course removing the internal secreting membrane of the cyst. This would be a natural protection, and I think that even the ligature can be suspended with. Why? If the cyst is broadly adherent to the peritoneum or intestine, or bladder, no one would cut through those parts. to separate the cyst, but, he would cut through the cyst wall, as I have done before myself, leaving that piece of the cyst which is attached to the other organ, remove the secreting membrane; often without any hemorrhage and without any bad consequences. This I will put into practice, as soon as I have the proper chance.

I have up to this time employed the intra-peritoneal method in every case. Now comes the most important duty: namely, to take time and search for every bleeding vessel, secure them by fine linen carbolized ligatures, cut short. You may have to use one only, you may have to employ 50 or 100, no matter how many, stop the bleeding, wash out the abdominal cavity, with the artifical serum, after this is done thoroughly, you are ready to close the wound. This you can do in different ways. Sometimes I take one of these large pins, put two of these beads upon it, then thrust it into the one side into the abdominal wall, an inch from the edge of the wound, and be careful to embrace skin, muscular and other tissuse, and the peritoneum, then let it run through the other side from within, out; using three or four of these pins, then bring the lips of the wound together, so that the peritoneal surfaces will meet (for this is important.) They unite within the first 24 hours. Then put two more beads upon each of the other side of the pin and fasten with thread or small pieces of lead, (these are deep seated sutures,) then I put in as many superficial linen sutures as may be needed to close the wound completely. Or I use strong silk or linen sutures for the deep seated ones instead of the pin. A double ligature is introduced as described, than insert through the loops on either side, a strip of strong piece of pasteboard, previously, well saturated in carbolized oil, and use like a quill suture. Oiled paper or glass is the only material I know of that does not irritate the skin. However, the pin and beads are preferable, for the reason, if any swelling takes place, one or more of the beads may be broken, and the tension relieved. I never use cat-gut, it absorbs too quickly, and is not safe. You may also employ the method I adopted in my last case, that is to close the peritoneum with fine ligatures in the manner I showed you previously in intestinal sutures, the rest is closed as usual, not inclosing the peritoneum.

I mentioned before, that it might be an advantage to cut through the rectus muslce, half or an inch beyond the Linea Albae, instead of directly throu.h it in the median line, and why? If the peritoineum is enclosed like an apron between the aponeurosis of the rectus muscle it might prevent the perfect union of the same and the patient is in danger of a ventral hernia afterwards. It never happened in any of my cases, but ventral hernia has been the sequel after ovariatomy, and it strikes me that this may be the cause. To avoid this, the method last described may be employed. But if the incision is made through the muscles, and union takes place, there can be no such a danger.

The wound being closed, everything cleaned, now comes the dressing. I use several layers of antiseptic gauze, over this a large layer of salicylic cotton, then a flannel bandage snugly applied. However, where the abdomen is flabby it is well to support the abdomen with one or two pieces of adhesive plaster, "mole skin" before applying the dressing. Then I generally give a hypodermic injection of 1-4 gr. of morphine.

Have all instruments and utensils brought out of the room before the patient rallies, leave her on the operating bed.

The after treatment depends upon circumstances, and must be adapted accordingly.

In regard to the p   time for operating see my article in the Cincinnati "Obstetric Gazette," March 1880.

For form of note book see Well's. Page 141. It is the one I adopted.

Now gentlemen, allow me one word in conclusion. You as experienced practitioners came here to gain that additional knowledge which will enable you to perform your duties more thoroughly, more faithfully, do not shrink from that duty, whenever you are called upon to give a human being the last chance the last hope.

I have tried to explain to you all the steps as well as possible. No doubt every one of you will feel more competent now, and have the courage to undertake the task. And I advise you to do it, when ever a chance presents itself to you. You often will hear a specialist say, no one but an expert should do this or that. Now I dislike such utterances and hate to read such sentences.

They can not live to be experts always, some one has to take their places, and how did they become experts? By practice.

But one thing I will say to you, and remind you of, and that is whatever operation you may undertake to perform, be well prepared, even into the smallest details, depend upon no one but yourself. Do not think that all those little matters are idle fancies of mine. They are necessary, no one will meet with success, unless he takes care of the minor things. Have everything on hand that may be needed, there is no earthly excuse for not having them, when they are within your reach, unless you are in the wilderness, then you may cut a reed, and use it for a tracer, or sharpen up a flint stone for a scalpel.

Give your patient all your time and attention until out of danger, the excuse of not having time is not justifiable. Do not accept a patient if you cannot attend to him properly. Be not guilty of any neglect. So that your conscience may be still and quiet, for omission is as censurable as commission.

I often remain with my patients 2 and 3 and 4 days, and nights at a time, By doing so I saved one of my patients, whose life otherwise would have faded away, before assistance could have been summoned.

When I first begun this operation 5 years ago, I had to bear a good deal of sarcasm, on account of the course I pursued. I stood it all, but to-day I am well satisfied.

This will finish my course of lectures. I thank you for your kind attention. I hope we shall meet again, and while I bid you a farewell.

    I remain
        Yours truly.

Edw. Borck.

225 WASHINGTON AVENUE.

A report of all cases of Ovariotory and Abdominal operations, performed by me since 1878, will appear in a near future in addition to those already reported.

Fracture of the femur, third edition, in preparation.

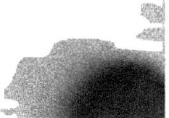

CPSIA information can be obtained
at www.ICGtesting.com
Printed in the USA
LVHW021244071118
596294LV00004B/780